Love, Life, and The Pursuit of Health

Love, Life, and The Pursuit of Health

Melissa Paquin

Love, Life, and The Pursuit of Health

Love, Life, and the Pursuit of Health

By Melissa Paquin

Paperback ISBN: 979-8-9950553-0-3

E-book ISBN: 979-8-9950553-1-0

Cover design cover image generated by ChatGPT using prompts from the author.

Printed in the United States of America

The Progenext Group, Hampton GA

An important note: This book is not intended as a substitute for the medical recommendation of physicians or other health-care providers. Rather, it is intended to offer information to help the reader cooperate with physicians and health professionals in a mutual quest for optimum well-being.

The identities of people described in the case histories have been changed to protect patient confidentiality.

The publisher and the author are not responsible for any goods and/or services offered or referred to in this book and expressly disclaim all liability in connection with the fulfillment of orders for any such goods and/or services and for any damage, loss, or expense to person or property arising out of or relating to them.

To my mother, who showed me what compassion in healthcare truly looks like, and whose dedication to nursing first inspired my love of medicine.

To the teachers, mentors, colleagues, and students who fueled my curiosity and deepened my respect for science.

To every patient who has ever felt confused, unheard, or overwhelmed within the healthcare system — this book is for you. May you always feel empowered to ask questions, seek understanding, and take your rightful place at the center of your own care.

And to my family and friends, whose constant encouragement and unwavering belief in me made these pages possible.

Here's to Love, Life, and the Pursuit of Health.

Love, Life, and The Pursuit of Health

A Guide to Taking Control of Your Health

In a world where medical information is abundant but often confusing, Dr. Melissa Paquin offers a refreshingly clear path to health autonomy. Drawing from her unique background in both healthcare genetics and education, she bridges the critical gap between what scientists discover, what healthcare providers understand, and what everyday people need to know.

Love, Life, and The Pursuit of Health is your essential guide to becoming an informed, empowered participant in your own healthcare. Dr. Paquin demystifies the complex healthcare system with accessible explanations of crucial topics: understanding the difference between doctors and other healthcare providers, developing health and genetic literacy, recognizing evidence-based practice, and navigating the promise of personalized medicine. She tackles difficult subjects like healthcare disparities and distinguishes real science from pseudoscience, equipping readers to make truly informed decisions.

This isn't about challenging your doctors, it's about understanding them. Dr. Paquin emphasizes that health autonomy means being an integral part of your healthcare journey, knowing when to trust medical professionals and when to ask for a second opinion. With real-world examples, plain-language medical glossaries, and practical advice, she shows that knowledge is the foundation of autonomy.

Whether you're managing a chronic condition, making decisions for dependents, or simply navigating annual checkups, this book empowers you to ask the right questions, understand the answers, and advocate for yourself with confidence. Dr. Paquin's passion for helping people shines through every page, making complex medical concepts accessible without oversimplifying.

Your health. Your life. Your informed choices. This book puts you back in the driver's seat.

Introduction: Let Me Introduce Myself

I have been a part of a medical family for my whole life. So much so that my first core memories are of my mother studying for her RN exam. Fast forward to my old(er) age and even now my very best friend is a brilliant registered nurse. I even ended up pursuing my degree under the School of Nursing at Clemson University. Suffice to say, I have been immersed in the world of medicine for a long time and have a passion for helping people.

Along with my lifelong love of medicine, I also have always loved science. The biological sciences in particular are my favorite discipline. I took extra science classes in high school, like the giant nerd I am, just to be able to learn more. The love of science only grew with me as I got older and led to multiple degrees in biology. My doctorate degree is the ultimate culmination of both loves since it is in Healthcare Genetics. It is also what gives me a unique perspective on both medicine and science.

I decided to write this book because I saw a significant gap between what scientists spend their lives doing, what healthcare professionals understand and what the everyday consumer knows. I have seen many people hurt by their own lack of knowledge and I figured the least I could do was try to bridge that gap. And voilà the idea for a book was born. My hope for everyone that reads this book is that they feel a little more empowered and confident when making healthcare decisions. If I can convince people to feel confident enough to ask pertinent questions about their healthcare, then the book has done its job.

Thank you to everyone who has taken the time to read my book. I hope that you enjoy reading it as much I enjoyed writing it. Here is to Love, Life and The Pursuit of Health!

Health Autonomy: My Health, My Choice

I want to start off by talking about health autonomy because it is the basis for everything else in the book. Health autonomy is the understanding that if you are capable of making decisions about your own health, care, and well-being then you have the right to do just that. If you have dependents (like children or adults that lack the ability to make their own choices) then this autonomy extends to them. Autonomy assumes that you have the ability to make your own choices and that you also have the understanding to make your own choices. So, this means that you understand the healthcare system, everything that the doctors tell you, all of your rights, etc. True autonomy requires knowledge.

Health autonomy is a foundational principle in modern healthcare, emphasizing the right and ability of individuals to make informed decisions about their own health and medical care. From treatment options and preventive measures to lifestyle choices and end-of-life care, health autonomy underlines respect for personal values, beliefs, and goals. As societies become more diverse and healthcare systems more complex, understanding and promoting health autonomy is both a moral imperative and a practical necessity.

At its core, health autonomy refers to the capacity and freedom of individuals to make choices about their own health, free from coercion or unwarranted interference. This concept is rooted in the ethical principle of respect for autonomy, one of the four pillars of biomedical ethics alongside beneficence, non-maleficence, and justice. Autonomy involves being able to understand information, appreciate the consequences of different choices, deliberate about options, and ultimately act in accordance with one's values and preferences.

Why is health autonomy important? Well, having autonomy in healthcare is very important for a number of reasons that are important for us as individuals as well as for the healthcare system in general. Firstly, everyone has the right to their own dignity and well-being. Believe it or not being afforded the opportunity to make your own health decisions affirms self worth and respect as an individual. It says that you are important and worthy of making your own decisions. Secondly, it is a way that can foster trust between individuals and the healthcare industry. If you feel like you are in control of your own health, you are more likely to trust medical professionals. This leads to an increase in positive health outcomes which basically means that if you trust that you have the ability to make decisions, you are more likely to seek treatment. Health autonomy also encourages people to be health literate, which we will cover in the next chapter. Finally, it is just plain ethically to allow people to make their own decisions about their own health. It is important to note that this does not mean you shouldn't listen to the medical professionals, it means that you should be a part of the decision-making process and have the ultimate say. This is why I cannot stress enough how important it is that you make INFORMED decisions, which are based on KNOWLEDGE.

At this point you are probably thinking to yourself that's great but what does that really mean and why do I care? Well, let me give you a few real-world examples to help you understand what I am talking about. Let's say that you are just a regular guy that needs a checkup with your primary care provider (PCP), so you make an appointment. During this appointment your PCP suggests that you receive this new vaccine since you are at risk for getting really sick. You are not generally against vaccines but you don't understand what this vaccine is for or how it works.

You have the right to ask your PCP to explain to you why you are more at risk for getting sick than other people, what the vaccine does, and how it works. You have a right to ask for what the potential side effects are and what the benefits are. Based off of what your PCP says you make the decision that the vaccine is not right for you.

Let's look at a different example. Let's say that you make another appointment with your PCP, again it is just a regular check-up. During this check-up up your PCP asks you a bunch of questions. Some of them are about your physical health and some of them are about your mental health. They may ask you questions about feeling unmotivated, lack of energy, sadness, etc. Your PCP suggests that you get on medication for depression. While this is something that you are open to, you are not comfortable with your PCP prescribing it for you since they are not an expert in mental health. So, you ask your PCP for a referral to a psychiatrist who can properly diagnose you as well as prescribe you medication if it is deemed necessary. In this scenario if the PCP agrees and gives you the recommendation then that is great. However, if they do not want to give you the recommendation then what? Well, you can fire them and find a new one.

What are some of the barriers to obtaining health autonomy? The largest barrier to attaining health autonomy is lack of knowledge. This includes not understanding complex medical terminology that is common to medical professionals. This doesn't mean that you have to go out and memorize a medical dictionary, but it does mean that you have to ask your medical professional to explain terms that are important to your care. Another barrier is medical paternalism which basically means that your doctor has a "god complex" and always thinks they know best. You can overcome this barrier by firing any medical professional that you don't feel like is listening to you. This doesn't mean that your doctor should always do what you ask but it does mean that your doctor treats you with dignity and respect. If you do not feel comfortable with your medical professional, you can change them or at the very least get a second opinion. In fact, second opinions are great for any major health decision and I highly recommend them. Systemic inequities are another barrier to health autonomy that we will discuss later in the book.

Basically, health autonomy is being an integral part of your own health journey. It is having enough knowledge to be able to ask questions and understand the answers. It is knowing when to trust the medical professionals and when to ask for a second opinion. It is important to mention again that health autonomy doesn't mean you know better than your medical professionals, it just means that you should be involved in all aspects of decision making. Every person deserves to be treated with dignity and respect when dealing with their health.

2

My Doctors Not A Doctor?

I am sure you see this title and think what the heck is she talking about now. Let us begin with talking about what it takes to be a medical doctor. Obviously, there are many years of college involved, including medical school and residency. This means that a person goes through four years of undergraduate college. After that they have to take a big test called the MCAT which will decide if they even can apply to medical schools. Then if they are accepted to medical school, it is another one to two years of intense instruction and three to four years of clinical rotation. Assuming that they pass, they then have to pass a licensing exam. After that these baby doctors have to apply for a residency program. Residency can last up to seven years depending on what they have chosen as their specialty. Obviously, doctors like surgeons will have a longer residency since it is a more intense specialty. After all of this doctors can now apply for a state license to practice medicine. If a doctor wishes to become a specialist then they may pursue a fellowship which can last an additional one to three years. Finally, a doctor may choose to become board certified in their specialty which means that they have to pass rigorous exams given by their peers to show that they are experts in their specialty. Not all doctors are board-certified because it is not a requirement to practice medicine.

Clearly, becoming a doctor is a long and arduous process. It takes a lot of skill and dedication to become a doctor. However, that does not mean that all doctors are created equally or that you are even seeing a doctor at all. For instance, primary care providers are not always medical doctors. This of course doesn't mean that they are not medical professionals, just that they are not doctors. Our healthcare system is leaning more towards having Nurse Practitioners and Physician's Assistants be our primary care providers as opposed to medical doctors. There is absolutely nothing wrong with having an NP or a PA take care of all the usual annual exam things, like physicals, vaccines and things like that. The rules about what NPs and PAs are able to do vary among the states. In states that offer full independence NPs can order tests and prescribe medications without the oversight of a medical doctor. However, the scope of the medications that they can order may be limited compared to a doctor. In states that have limited or restricted care NPs have to practice under the license of a medical doctor and cannot practice independently. PAs are very similar to NPs; they just follow different models when schooling.

Having an NP or PA as a primary care provider makes sense in a lot of ways. For one, the cost of becoming an NP or PA is significantly less than becoming a medical doctor. This means that they are able to make more money sooner without having a specialty. Especially in states where they are allowed to work independently, NPs have filled the need left from provider shortages. NPs also tend to have shorter wait times and more accessibility. NPs and PAs can also be a part of specialty practices where they work under medical doctors. While it is great that these kinds of providers are filling a gap for primary care, it is important to note that they have not undergone the aforementioned extensive training to become a medical doctor. This means that their scope of practice is limited and that they are not doctors.

Another thing that makes doctors unequal is specialization. I mentioned before that after medical school doctors can elect to further their education with a specialization. This is where you get cardiologists (heart doctors), neurologists (anything to do with the brain and nervous system), psychiatrists (deals with mental health), basically every organ system has its own specialist. These doctors train after traditional medical school in their particular specialty and may even continue to become board-certified. If a doctor is board-certified, that means that they have proven themselves in front of a board of experts in their field of medicine. So, what does this mean to you? Let's start with the role of the primary care provider which is routine care. This includes things like annual physicals, vaccines, refilling prescriptions and most importantly giving referrals.

Ok, so why are referrals important? Well, referrals are usually required by your insurance company so that you can see a specialist. Even if your insurance company doesn't require a referral, the specialist usually wants you to have a referral. Your primary care provider is the one that will provide you with a referral. It is your PCPs job to send out these referrals to a specialist; it is not their job to be the specialist. For example, you would not call an electrician if you needed a plumber, would you? So why would you want a doctor who is not a specialist to treat you? If you have symptoms of depression and anxiety, you need a psychiatrist. Mental health is a specialization that can be very complex, especially in children and young adults. Diagnosing mental health issues can be tricky and treating them is even trickier. So, if your PCP wants to just give you some pills for your depression, that might not be the best course of action. It would make more sense for the provider to recommend a psychiatrist and probably a therapist.

In the same vein if your PCP does bloodwork that shows that you have estimated glomerular filtration rates (eGFR) that are lower than average. You are probably thinking, what the heck does that mean and in all honesty, it doesn't matter because that's not the point. However, suffice to say it has to do with your kidney function and a low eGFR can be an indicator of kidney failure. Now let's say that your PCP orders the bloodwork, sees that your eGFR is lower than average and tells you such. Let us also say that your PCP does not recommend that you go see a nephrologist (kidney doctor) or even a urologist (urinary tract doctor) but just tells you to not take so many NSAIDS (Ibuprofen, Aleve, etc.). How would you feel about that? Would you feel comfortable not having your levels explained to you, other testing done, or having a doctor who is not specializing in your kidneys to determine your treatment options? Again, I say if your toilet is actively overflowing, would you want an electrician to come and tell you that it is overflowing or would you like a plumber to come and fix the actual problem? I think we would all agree we would prefer the toilet water to stay in the toilet. Just as it is preferable that doctors stay in their area of expertise.

Therefore, doctors are not all created equally and they have specializations. This is part of why autonomy is important. You can tell your doctor that you want a second opinion, or you can tell them that you want a referral. PCPs are great resources and they have a great ability to manage medicines. However, they should recognize when you need a specialist and you should be able to ask for a referral. Same goes for Nurse Practitioners and for Physician assistants, excellent resources but they are not doctors.

3

If My Doctors Not A Doctor: What Is He?

O k, so we already started talking about how your primary care provider is not necessarily a doctor (hence PCP meaning primary care *provider* and not physician). Let us now take a look at other professionals that sometimes get confused with medical doctors. Now, I want to preface this by saying I am not disparaging anyone's profession but remember with autonomy comes knowledge. Therefore, people need to know what professionals do and what their scope of practice is.

Let's start with chiropractors. Chiropractors can call themselves "doctor" but they in no way are medical doctors. Chiropractors receive a Doctor of Chiropractic terminal degree and pass a 4-part national board exam. There are also specific state requirements that each chiropractor has to meet in order to maintain their licensure. The chiropractic curriculum does have basic science classes including biochemistry and anatomy. However, they are not medically trained and more specifically are not trained in pathophysiology (all about diseases). Your chiropractor is allowed to take x-rays but this not necessarily as a diagnostic tool but more so to make sure they are not causing damage. A chiropractor should not be making diagnoses or planning treatments for anything not related to body structure. Even then, seeing a medical doctor is still advised because they have more education and access to diagnostic tools like MRIs.

Next on the list are physical therapists. Physical therapy is generally the first course of treatment for most injuries. Physical therapists receive a Doctor of Physical Therapy degree but again, it is not medical degree. Similar to the chiropractors, physical therapists also have to pass a licensure exam. Again like a chiropractor, physical therapy school focuses a lot on movement and anatomy. Although physical therapists can help to diagnose movement and functional issues, they should not be diagnosing medical conditions. As a matter of fact physical therapists generally need a referral from a medical doctor in order to get paid by insurance companies. Occupational therapists are similar to physical therapists but they focus on skills that are necessary for everyday living. This includes things like getting dressed, eating, doing school or going to work. Occupational therapists work with people who have physical, emotional or mental disabilities that make it difficult to perform everyday tasks. Occupational therapists have to obtain a master's degree and have specific licensure requirements depending on the state they practice in. Once again occupational therapists are not medical doctors. Another type of therapist is a speech language pathologist commonly known as a speech therapist. Again, they have a master's degree and have different licensure requirements depending on the state. SLPs can diagnose speech and language disorders and swallowing disorders. They work with people of all ages that have different communication disorders. For instance, they will help young children who have stuttering issues or tongue ties. However, they are still not a medical doctor.

Let us move on to your vision. Most people don't know that there is a difference between an optometrist and an ophthalmologist. An optometrist is the person you go to for all your annual vision tests and they are the ones that give you a prescription for contacts and glasses. And although optometrists receive a Doctor of Optometry degree, once again they are not medical doctors. They are able to diagnose early signs of eye disease and also prescribe some medications, they are still not medical doctors. Ophthalmologists on the other hand, have gone to medical school and are medical doctors that have specialized in the eye. They can do all the things that optometrists can but they can also perform surgery for things like cataracts or LASIK and treat complex diseases and disorders. You can go to see an ophthalmologist for routine visits but you cannot see an optometrist for LASIK surgery.

While I cannot go over every profession that people get confused with medical doctors, I do think it is important to go over professionals that deal with mental health. There are a number of different professionals that people see for various mental health reasons. The first and most common is a therapist. A therapist is a broad term that can include counselors, psychologists, social workers and others that provide therapy. All therapists have to be licensed but the extent and scope of practice depends on which license they possess. Now a therapist is not the same thing as a counselor although they both can be resources to reach mental health goals. A counselor is a certified professional that help people attain short term goals. For instance, a substance abuse counselor can help someone recover from addiction. Counselors are certified by different organizations based on their specializations. Counselors have some ability to diagnose but it varies by state and is limited. Ok, back to therapists. A master's degree level therapist include family and marriage therapists or clinical licensed social workers and focus mostly on mental health treatments. Training between all types of master level trained therapist varies immensely. A psychologist is a doctoral level therapist who is not a medical doctor. Psychologists delve more deeply into the science behind mental disorders. Psychologists are more likely to treat more severe mental illnesses and also can be researchers. Psychiatrists are medical doctors and they are the only mental health professionals that can prescribe medications. Most of the time it is a good idea to see both a therapist and a psychiatrist to help treat all aspects of mental illness. Now life coaches are not therapists at all and are not regulated in any way. Anyone with a couple of bucks can become a life coach.

Long story short is that there are a lot of professionals that people confuse with medical doctors. All professionals have their place and can be important. However, it is an integral part of health autonomy to understand these differences. Everyone has the right to see a chiropractor if they want to but you also have to know what a chiropractor can do and what they cannot. The same goes for an optometrist or a physical therapist. Part of healthcare autonomy is understanding what each professional is capable of doing and who you need to see when.

4

Health Literacy: Wait I know How To Read!

A key component to health autonomy is health literacy. I am sure you read that sentence and think, wait you think I can't read???!! If you have chosen to pick up this book, then I am positive that you can read but I am not positive that you necessarily understand your health information. So, what is health literacy exactly? Well before you can make informed healthcare decisions, IE have autonomy, you have to be *informed.* That is where the literacy part comes in, it is obtaining, understanding, and using health related information to make decisions. You have to have the information in order to be able to make decisions based *off* the information. Basically, you cannot use what you do not know. Health literacy is the knowing part so that way you have the information necessary to make important healthcare decisions.

The first part of gaining knowledge is to know where to get the information. Just like we talked about how not all doctors are created equal, not all sources of information are created equal either. It is important to know who is giving the information and what they have to gain from providing the information. The most obvious place to get health related information is your primary care provider. They are a great place to ask questions and explore options, especially if it is regarding things like vaccines. However, they may not have the answers that you need so if this is case then where do you go?

Another great source of information is the National Institutes of Health (NIH). The NIH is a collection of agencies that promote and fund biomedical and health research. Now, this is the part of where some of you may say well all researchers care about is big pharma or making millions of dollars. As someone who is a scientist and has been among scientists for a long time, I can tell you that most researchers are not making a lot of money and are not in it for the glory. Becoming a researcher is also a long and arduous process that takes many years to complete. After completion many researchers are all competing for the same grant money which does not make the researchers rich. A lot of researchers end up as professors in academic institutions where they have to split their time between teaching and performing their research. If you have ever been to college, you know that most of your professors do not make a lot of money. Long story short is that most scientists are not in the game for the money, they are in it because they love science and want to help people. The NIH is responsible for funding some of the major health related research and also for providing access to health-related information. It is an excellent source of scientific publications but it also has links to information that is easier to understand.

There are also a number of websites that are dedicated to promoting health literacy. Medline plus is a site that has tutorials and a drug encyclopedia geared towards helping everyday people better understand their health. There are also body part or disease specifics organizations that have informative websites. The American Heart Association has all sorts of information on heart health. The National Kidney Foundation has information on kidney health and resources for those who have chronic kidney disease. You can also go to your local medical universities website and they will have information as well. If you have a chronic disease there are a lot of advocacy groups that have information related to your specific disease.

A really basic step that all people can do to improve their health literacy is to learn everyday medical terms. Understanding the difference between chronic and acute or hereditary and genetic will help you to better understand your medical conditions. To help you get started, I have provided a glossary of terms at the end of this book. You do not have to be a scholar to understand basic medical terminology and it will help you understand aftercare instructions, consent forms, and diagnoses. It will also help you to use the resources that we spoke about above, if you have some basic terms down you can better understand the information presented by the NIH or Medline Plus.

No matter where you get your health information from it is very important that you are able to assess the credibility of the source and the relevance to your situation. If the Covid epidemic showed us anything it is that people will make up information when they don't have any information. Therefore, it is really important that you know where your information is coming from and what they have to gain from sharing this information. When you are reading scientific articles, you can see if the researchers have conflicts of interest and if the article is published in a peer reviewed journal. Researchers do not get paid to publish their work and it is generally frowned upon to pay to publish.

Tiktok and other social media platforms can be great sources of information but they also can be great sources of *mis*information. Anyone with a PhD, MD, EdD, PsyD, JD, etc can call themselves doctor. This means that you could be getting health information from someone calling themselves "doctor" but really they are a glorified gym teacher or a businessman or even a lawyer. It is important to know who is giving you the information, what kind of professional are they? Are they respected in their field? Are they selling products or propaganda of some sort? How did they gain their knowledge? It is really important to always take the information you find on the internet with a grain of salt and to verify what the Tiktoker is telling you with other sources of information. Trust but verify is a great motto to live by.

Now that you have gathered as much information as you can, the next part of health literacy is using this information. Use the information you have gained to ask questions and to get clarification from your provider. Health literacy helps to improve communication between providers and their patients. It helps you as a patient make more informed decisions about treatment options and medications which directly leads to increased health autonomy. Keep in mind, I do not think having increased health literacy means you know more than trained professionals, I think that it means you have increased ability to ask questions and make informed decisions.

5

Genetic Literacy: What The Heck Is That?

Now that we have talked about health literacy in general, I would like to talk about genetic literacy specifically. The Covid epidemic showed me that genetics are vastly misunderstood and yet are something that *need to* be understood. Genetic literacy is your ability to understand genetics; what are genetics, how they influence your health, and how they shape medicine. Genetic literacy is important in making informed medical treatment decisions, understanding genetic testing, and knowing your right to genetic privacy.

What are genetics and why do we care? Genetics is anything to do with genes, traits, and heredity. Genomics is a fancy way of saying anything to do with all your genes and how they work and interact. Your genes are the blueprint for your body, they provide the instructions for all the structures and functions that take place in your body. Everything that happens in your body starts with your genes. Now it is important to mention that there are a lot of factors that play into gene expression and many of them are too complicated for this book. I am not saying that it is important that you become an expert in genetics but what I am saying is that you have to know enough to at least be able to ask the right questions.

So what role does genetics play in your health? The first role starts before birth. There is carrier screening which is when neither you nor your partner have the disease but you are tested to see if either of you are carriers of the gene. Diseases like cystic fibrosis require a "bad" copy from both the mom and the dad in order for the child to have the disease. Prenatal screening can see if you and your partner are carriers of any genes that in combination may cause your child to have the disease. This is not an all encompassing test, which means that they are not going to be able to test for all the diseases, but the most common. The next genetic testing happens during pregnancy for things like downs syndrome or trisomy 13 which where there is an extra copy of chromosome 13 leading to high rates of miscarriage and still births. After birth the baby can be genetically tested for a large panel of genetic disorders that are usually treatable. Later on in life genetic testing can be used for diagnostics for diseases like Hunting's Disease, Polycystic Kidney Disease and many others. Being able to properly identify diseases correctly and early can drastically effect prognosis, depending on the disease of course.

Genetics are also used for predictive testing like with *BRCA1* and *BRCA2* genes and breast cancer. If an individual has a specific *BRCA1* or *BRCA2* gene mutation their risk of getting breast or ovarian cancer is higher when compared to those who do not have those mutations. Another common predictive test is for colorectal cancer. Another example would be for familial hypercholesterolemia which indicates a higher risk for high cholesterol. There is also a test for long QT syndrome which is a heart condition. It is important to note that a positive predictive test only indicates an increased risk of getting the disease. The risk rate depends on the disease, the gene and other risk factors. Just because you have a positive predictive test does not mean you will get the disease and a negative one also doesn't mean you definitely will not get the disease. Again it all depends on the disease, genes and other risk factors. However, knowing that you have an increased risk can increase prophylactic care, help you to reduce other risk factors that are in your control, and increase surveillance.

Another relatively unknown use of genetic testing is pharmacogenomics. This is how your particular genetic make up will affect certain medications. This is important because it can optimize drug therapy, meaning that it can help ensure you get the medication that will work at the right dose the first time. It is also helpful to minimize adverse effects or side effects. This is a big step towards personalized medicine which is what we will talk about in a subsequent chapter. So what is pharmacogenomics exactly? The genes in each of your cells has a blueprint that determines how drugs are metabolized (basically how fast they go from an active form to an inactive form), how they are transported, and what their targets are in the body. For example some people have a gene that means that they need a higher dose of certain drugs because they are what we call fast metabolizers. This means that they have the gene that makes the drugs go from an active to an inactive form quickly. So they will need a higher dose of certain drugs.

There are a number of ways that pharmacogenomics are being used currently. One way is in cancer treatment drugs. Many cancer treatments are tailored both to the patients particular genome as well as to the tumors genome. This just means that testing will be done to see if the drug treatments will be effective based on your genes and the genes in your tumor. Another way it is used is in mental health medications. Pharmacogenomics can be used to determine what antidepressants or antipsychotics will work for you based on your genetics. It can also be used to determine what blood thinners at what dosage will work for you. Long story short pharmacogenomics is key for personalized medicine and takes a lot of the guess work out of medication choices and dosages.

Another component of genetic literacy is having a basic understanding of things like DNA and RNA and how they affect treatment options. I will give some examples here but if you want an in-depth explanation, book a seminar. One of the big things about genes and your health is gene therapy. Gene therapy is too complex a topic for this book, however I can give a brief overview of the important parts. Gene therapy includes things like replacing a faulty copy of a gene with one that is functioning. Another example of gene therapy is adding a gene into the genome that works not by replacing the one that doesn't but in addition to the one that does not. The opposite can be done with gene silencing where gene expression is inhibited (stopped) so that harmful proteins are not made. Lastly, gene therapy can be used to promote apoptosis (programmed cell death) in cancer cells. Another example is replacing faulty genes in people with Duchene's Muscular Dystrophy with working ones. This can be done by using vectors like viruses that carry the gene into the cell and replace it or by taking out the cells and replacing the gene "in vitro".

Genetics also plays a role in disease prevention such as with vaccines. DNA is the cell's blueprint and mRNA is the cells translator. mRNA takes the information from the DNA and moves it to the part of the cell that will actually make the protein that the blueprint codes for. For example mRNA vaccines don't use actual viruses to invoke an immune response. Instead they use mRNA which is a code for making a particular protein that will invoke the immune response. Basically they instruct our own cells to make the part of the pathogen (disease causing thing) that our immune system will remember and fight off when it comes in contact with it again. mRNA is not designed to stay in the body and therefore the body will destroy it. mRNA technology is currently being studied to help treat many diseases and even creating a cancer vaccine. The future of mRNA technology and the treatment of disease is very promising but also misunderstood.

Another important aspect of genetic literacy is understanding your rights. GINA is the Genetic Information Nondiscrimination Act and was put in place in the early 2000s to protect individual's genetic information. GINA was put in place so that health insurance companies cannot use your genetic information to determine premiums, eligibility or deny coverage due to "pre-existing" conditions. This protection only extends to health insurance and doesn't include disability, life or long-term care insurance. Similarly, GINA protects employees from being discriminated against by employers based on their genetic information. Now it is important to note that if you use a genetic screening company for ancestry or other reasons, you very well may be signing a clause that states they can sell or use your genetic information for research purposes. This is not the same as using your genetic information to determine employment or health insurance coverage. Always read the fine print on anything you sign to make sure it is something that you are comfortable with.

Again, it is not important that you become a genetics expert but it is important that you have enough knowledge to ask appropriate questions. Genetics play an important role in every part of your health, from disease manifestation to treatments. Genetics will also continue to play a very important role in personalized medicine. You need to ask questions when you do not understand something and then make sure you don't stop until you get it.

6

Evidence Based Practice: What am I, A Lawyer?

What is evidence based practice and what does it have to do with health autonomy? Evidence based practice is when healthcare providers combine the most current research, their clinical expertise, and your own personal preferences to tailor the best care possible. Really it is the combining of traditional bench science, which is the scientist who are doing the research on disease, and everyday medicine. If the results of research are not being put into practice, then what is the point of the research? Evidence based practice includes asking clear clinical questions that directly relate to your needs as a patient. After the question has been formulated, the next step is looking through peer reviewed research to find the answer to the question. This means looking at sources that have been validated and includes the research that we mentioned previously. Next it is important to apply the knowledge learned to the current situation. This is the step where the healthcare professional will bring the treatment plan or whatnot to you and ask what your thoughts and feelings are. The last step is assessing the process and seeing what can be improved for the next patient.

An example of evidence based practice is implementing a nurse led protocol to prevent bed sores in patients. Firstly, nurses identified that there was a high rate of bed sores in patients that were in the hospital in for long periods of time. So the nurses reviewed the most current research on how to help prevent bed sores in patients that stay in the hospital for long periods of time. The research that they found stated that turning patients every 2 hours and using specialized mattresses would reduce the risk of these patients' getting bedsores. The nurses then took what they learned and created protocols to implement that would help prevent bed sores. After a certain period of time the nurses came back and see if the protocols are working. It is found that these protocols are reducing the rate of bed sores so now it becomes standard practice. Now this is an example of how evidence based practice protocols are created but obviously, health professionals are not developing new protocols for each patient.

Ok, so lets look at an example that is something you may come across. Suppose that you or a family member has been having some pretty bad knee pain. You go to the doctor and they tell you that you have osteoarthritis of your knee. You also know that you have a history of moderate high blood pressure and you have heard that NSAIDs (like ibuprofen) can cause problems if they are taken for long periods of time. The doctor suggests to you that there is a new medication called COX-2 inhibitors that can reduce the pain in your knee without causing the issues that long term NSAID can. The doctor then shows you that there is research that backs up that COX-2 inhibitors can reduce knee pain and reduce the risk of side effects. That is evidence based practice in real life. Of course it is dependent upon the healthcare provider to be up to date on the current research so that they can provide this information to you. But you can also ask for the most current information on whatever it is that is bringing you to the doctor.

What are the benefits of evidence based practice and what does it have to do with health autonomy? The most obvious benefit is that it provides patients with the most up to date treatment options available. If we are assuming that the healthcare providers are reading the current research then that means they are providing you with the newest and most relevant care. In theory evidence based practice should also limit unnecessary procedures or treatments that don't work or are outdated. Evidence based practice also should reduce healthcare costs by reducing outdated and ineffective treatments. It also ensures that your health-care provider is continually learning and is up to date with the latest treatment options available. You are not the only one that should be constantly learning about health and healthcare options, your provider should also be constantly learning.

Speaking of using research to enhance medicine, I want to take a moment to talk about the researchers themselves. There are a lot of misconceptions around researchers, their access to funds and their intentions. Researchers dedicate their lives to their scientific discipline starting with the many years of school that it takes to become a researcher. No one goes into science because they want to be rich and famous. They go into science for the love of science and knowledge. There are only a few ways that researchers can get the money they need to conduct the research that will help to advance medicine. Really most money comes from grants which can be from the government or private organizations. Even researchers that work in academia (colleges and universities) are still dependent on grants to do their research. Basically all researchers are fighting for the same money out of the same pot. So the research that is going to help the most people is usually the one that is going to win the money. Which means that the more rare diseases and disorders are going to have more trouble getting funding which makes it harder to come up with treatment options. Why does any of this matter? Well it matters because the researchers are the ones that are coming up with the evidence for the evidence-based practice. Understanding where they get their money from and how that dictates what research can be conducted gives you a better understanding of evidence-based practice.

7

Personalized Medicine: You Are The Star

All of the topics we have covered so far are directly related to personalized medicine or precision medicine. Personalized medicine is when medicine is tailored to the individual and is not a one size fits all mentality. Personalized medicine considers genetic makeup, environment, lifestyle and other factors prevent, diagnose, and treat diseases. The biggest part of personalized medicine is understanding an individual's genetic makeup and the role it plays in healthcare. We talked about how genetic testing can determine your risk of developing disease. Well in personalized medicine your healthcare providers would look at your risk of developing breast cancer based off your *BRCA* gene variations, familial history, and other risk factors to determine your personal risk of developing breast cancer. Lets say that after looking at all the risk factors the doctor says that you have a very high chance of getting breast cancer at a young age. The doctor may then recommend personalized prophylactic care like increased monitoring (getting mammograms more often) or even a mastectomy with reconstructive surgery to reduce your risk of developing cancer. Now if the opposite scenario were to take place where the doctor says you have a lower risk of developing breast cancer based off the risk factors, they probably would not recommend additional prophylactic care. This in a nutshell is personalized medicine, where individuals get medical care based of their individual needs.

Biomarkers are another biological tool that can be used in personalized medicine. Biomarkers are biological substances found in your body that help to monitor biological processes. One example would be blood glucose (sugar) or cholesterol levels that can help determine if you have diabetes or heart problems. Biomarkers can also include things like blood pressure and body temperature. Biomarkers can be used to determine presence or absence of a disease, as in the case of blood sugars. They are used to determine if the person is at risk of getting a disease. For instance, if a man has high PSA levels they likely have prostate cancer. Biomarkers can also be used to determine if a person has a disease They can also be used to determine how treatments are working and if additional treatment options are needed. For instance, in our breast cancer example, biomarkers can be used after mastectomy to see if chemotherapy is needed or not. They also can be used to determine if a disease has gotten better, worse or has remained unchanged. Lastly, biomarkers can be used to determine if a person is even able to have certain treatments. Again if we use the breast cancer example, kidney biomarkers may be used to make sure that the person has healthy enough kidneys to receive chemotherapy.

Personalized medicine improves treatment outcomes by tailoring medicine to each individual. If you look at the persons genetic makeup, biomarkers, risk factors, environmental factors and beliefs then you can better choose a treatment plan that will have the most success. Tailoring treatment options to the individual instead of just giving general treatments also helps to reduce the side effects and adverse reactions to treatments. Making sure that medicine is personalized helps to use healthcare resources more efficiently as compared to trying general options first. Lastly and maybe most importantly is that personalized medicine allows you as the patient to make informed health decisions: Which we have said is a critical part of health autonomy. Overall, personalized medicine represents a shift toward more individualized, effective, and proactive healthcare, offering the promise of better health outcomes for patients.

8

Disparities: You Mean The System Is Not Perfect?

Disparities in healthcare refer to differences in access, quality, and outcomes of medical services among various groups within a population. Basically this means that different people have different access, quality, and outcomes in relation to their healthcare based on their race/ethnicity, socioeconomic status (how much money you have), where you live, and/or gender. This doesn't mean that the system is specifically designed to discriminate against people and it definitely doesn't meant that the healthcare providers are bad people. There are many factors that contribute to healthcare disparities including biases that the patient has themselves.

In general racial minorities and poor people are facing higher rates of chronic diseases, preventable diseases and overall poor health outcomes. There are a lot of reasons why this occurs. The most obvious reason is that there is a lack of access to preventative care. Especially if you have a lower income, going to the doctor when you are healthy is really not on your radar. A lack of proper education on why preventative medicine is important is also a key reason why certain populations are at a greater risk. There is also a lack of availability of care depending on the population and area that the population lives in. Outside of the city there is not as many doctors available as compared to bigger cities.

Another aspect of healthcare disparities is healthcare inequities. Inequities are unfair but avoidable differences in healthcare that lead to differing health outcomes in different groups of people. Again, I want to stress that even though these differences are avoidable it doesn't mean that they are on purpose. Every person has innate biases that shape their view of the world and the people that are in it, including healthcare professionals. These are deeply ingrained in our thought process and so that they become a natural part of our thinking. These inequities are not just limited to race or ethnicity but can extend to a number of different populations. Let us say that you have a history of depression and anxiety. However, these mental health conditions are perfectly controlled by your psychiatrist and therapist. You wake up one day and feel like your heart is beating funny so you decide to go to the doctor. The doctor looks at your medications and mental health history and decides that your heart feels funny because you are anxious. The doctor is exhibiting an innate bias towards people who have mental health issues. This doesn't mean that the doctor is a bad guy who hates depressed people, it just means that he has been conditioned to see people who have mental health issues in a certain way. However, this bias and inequity can lead to you not getting the proper care you need.

The effects of disparities in healthcare are far-reaching. Individuals from disadvantaged groups often experience higher rates of chronic diseases, lower life expectancy, increased hospitalizations, and poorer mental health. Disparities also contribute to greater healthcare costs and strain on public health systems. This basically means that more people get sicker and that because more people are sick, the cost of care also increases. I am not saying that all professionals are bad, there are lots really great healthcare professionals who treat all patients with dignity and respect. Even in my example above, I am not trying to say that the doctor is incompetent or a bad person. What I am saying is that disparities are another big reason why health autonomy is so important. It is crucial that you are able to stand up for yourself in an educated way.

9

Pseudoscience: Fake Science Not Fake News

This is the time that we take a moment to talk about what exactly science is. You may be thinking, why do I even care and what does this have to do with healthcare autonomy? Well considering that medicine is deemed medical science, it is quite relevant. Plus in order to be truly informed or autonomous you have to be able to distinguish between good information and bad information. This is why you need to know what is based on science and what is not. There is a lot of health information that is disguises itself as scientific but is really pseudoscience. This is nothing new, snake oil salesmen have been around since the dawn of time and are still here in the 21st century.

What is science? Science at its core is merely humans trying to understand the world around them. Science starts with making an observation, Sir Isaac Newton got hit on the head by an apple falling out of a tree and wondered why. Antibiotics were discovered when a petri dish was left out in the open and Alexander Flemming saw that the bacteria did not grow where there was mold (observation). Even today science begins with observation, it may look a little different then the past but it is still the same idea. Once an observation has been the next step is to ask a question that you want to answer based on that observation. Newton would ask something like why did the apple fall down and not float away. Flemming would say something like what killed the bacteria in that particular part of the petri dish and why did the rest survive. The next part is to create a hypothesis, which basically is an educated guess that is going to answer the question based on your observation.

I am sure when you hear the word "guess" you are already thinking what is the point of learning the difference between science and pseudoscience if any of it involves guessing. BUT it is not really a guess at all, that is just something that people say to get out of explaining the process. It actually takes literature reviews and a basic understanding of the question you are asking in order to make a hypothesis. So basically you have to do research before you can do your research to see if your research is even doable. Yes, that is a lot of work before the experiment can even be done. Once a hypothesis is formed the next part is to design an experiment that will test your hypothesis. This is how you will be able to decide to either accept or reject your hypothesis which just means you figure out if your answer is right or wrong. The type of experiment that is created really depends on the question that you are trying to answer. But that is too much to go into for our purposes here. After the experiment (whatever it may be) is complete, now it is time to analyze the results. This is definitely too complicated for the scope of this book but it is important to note that analyzing takes a lot of time and effort. It is also important to note that true scientist are not necessarily interested in being right (accepting their hypothesis), they really just want to learn about their observation. This whole process is known as the scientific method and has been around in some capacity for thousands of years. Scientist have always been pretty smart and they knew that there had to be some kind of process to keep science consistent. Hence the scientific method was developed and is consistently utilized.

Now you may be thinking this is it, it is all over. But alas it is not and that is actually a good thing. After all the questions, guesses, experiments, and analyzes, it is now time to validate the study. In modern times scientists are validated by being published in reputable journals, this is where everything starts to make sense (IE why I have included this chapter in this particular book and have made you suffer through the scientific method). These journals are where other scientists that are experts in their fields (and the field that the new experiment is in) decide if the new experiment has been done properly (if the scientists performing the experiment have any special interest), like getting paid by people who would benefit from a specific result, and if the results are valid. Part of this process is making sure that the study is reproducible, which is why the scientific method is so very important. It shows that any other scientist can follow the same procedure and should come up with the same results. This is a very a critical aspect of the scientific process, it is what keeps science consistent and honest. While we are on this topic, I think this is the time we should revisit how scientists make their money.

Scientists do not get paid a lot of money to conduct their research, we have talked about this before but here is where we go into details. There is basically one big pot of gold also known as grant money that most scientists have to get their funding from. Without going into how hard it is to even get this money, lets just suppose that we have gotten the grant. Does all that money just go to the researcher or the research? In fact it absolutely does not. From the grant the first 40% goes back to the institution (a lot of times this is a college but it can be other things), so right off the bat the researcher is only working with 60% of the funds. From that 60% the researcher has to pay themselves and everyone else that the grant stipulates. Then any expenses that have to do with the research are taken out of the grant, equipment, any incentives (like the ones you get for clinical trials or survey participation etc.), any thing that has to do with the research. It costs a lot to conduct one research study and chances are there will have to be multiple in order to answer even part of your question. Bottom line is that researchers are not making millions off of their research. Most research studies take *years* to complete and the researchers are probably not making any more than you and your family. Keep this in mind as you keep reading this chapter and the next time you say "why haven't they had a cure for this or why don't they know about this", remember who they is. They is the researchers in case that was unclear.

Ok, we have talked about what science is now is the time to discuss what pseudoscience and how it affects health autonomy. Pseudoscience is simply anything that says that it is science but does not follow the scientific method. Which means that maybe they only focus on the one thing that supports their claim but not the other things that contradict the claim. Or they have claims without any evidence at all. Pseudoscience does not follow the scientific method and most certainly does not go through a rigorous peer review process. At this point I hope you are saying to yourself, well what is an example so I can stay away? The biggest pseudoscience in healthcare is weight loss products, there is always a new pill to take or substance to ingest that will make you lose weight fast that has no proof whatsoever. Another example is homeopathy which should not be confused with holistic medicine.

Homeopathy at its root is "like cures like" meaning whatever is causing the issue can also cure the issue. There is no scientific base to homeopathic remedies and the results are subjective which means that the person taking the treatment is the one deciding if it is working. If we are honest, people can convince themselves that anything is working especially if they are not feeling well. Matter of fact a lot of homeopathic remedies have been proven to be false when actual science is involved. Not only is homeopathy pseudoscience but it is also unregulated which means that no one is checking these substances or "cures" to see if they make you sicker or if they interfere with other medicines or even other homeopathic substances. There is no basis for the claims of homeopathy other than "old wives tails" and something my mother used to do... There are a lot of examples of homeopathy, essential oils, red onions being used for hay fever, all sorts of things.

Another example of pseudoscience is controversial and that is antivaccination. Now I want to be clear in saying that understanding what vaccines are, how they work and why they are important and choosing not to vaccinate with every vaccination available, is not what I am talking about. I am talking about trying to create associations with diseases and vaccines that are not actually scientific. In science we say that correlation does not mean causation which simply means just because two things are true and may even be found together does not mean that one is the reason another happens. A very glaring example of this is the assertion that vaccination some how causes autism. This claim has been disproven time and time again in the scientific community but yet some people still believe it to be true. This is a good time to talk about what vaccinations really are. The whole point of a vaccine is to elicit an immune response so that your body is prepared when it meets the germ in real life. Nothing in a vaccine has the part of the germ (termed a pathogen) that can make you get the actual illness. Yes, you will feel some symptoms but as I said that is because the whole point of a vaccine is to make your body react like it has been infected. Vaccines can be made of the non-infectious parts of a germ, a dead germ, or a genetic sequence that tells our own bodies to make a piece of the germ that our body will recognize (mRNA). Vaccines have been around since 1796 and they have saved countless lives. This whole book is designed to give you autonomy over your health, in that spirit I cannot tell you what you should or shouldn't do in terms of your health which includes vaccination. What I can say is that I have attempted to show what is science and in that hope you make an informed decision.

Now let us talk about holistic medicine. Holistic medicine and homeopathy are not the same thing. As a matter of fact holistic medicine is very similar to personalized medicine. Holistic medicine aims to treat the person as a whole. This includes nutrition, traditional medicine, life style changes, anything that could contribute to the patients current condition. For example if you come into the doctors office for a headache, a non-holistic approach would be to just tell you to take an aspirin and go home. A holistic approach would be to ask about your diet, stress, activity levels, sleep schedule etc. to determine why you are having headaches. This does not mean that you still will not receive some sort of medicine for your headaches, it just means that it looks at you as a whole person (hence holistic).

I told you to remember that researchers do not make a lot of money off their research. Homeopathy is a *MULTIBILLION* dollar business, this is all profit since they don't have to worry about the pesky scientific method or actual evidence based practice. Hey if you love your essential oils then go for it but all I am saying is who is profiting off of you? It is certainly not the scientists who spend their lives trying to figure out all those answers that we talked about earlier. Another interesting example of pseudoscience goes back to a profession we discussed earlier, chiropractics. Now don't get all upset and stop reading. I am not saying that all chiropractors are charlatans or anything HOWEVER if they are telling you that they can cure your asthma (an autoimmune disorder) with an adjustment then you should definitely be wary. Have you ever noticed that those shady personal injury lawyers always recommend going to a particular chiropractor, again that is a red flag. You really have to look at who stands to make money and how much they are going to make off of selling you treatments, remedies, oils, etc.

Why does any of this matter? Well, if you remember the chapter on healthcare literacy I told you that you need to know what a credible source is. A credible source is a *scientific* one. It is one that goes through the scientific method and has been scrutinized by experts in the scientific community. The discoveries are published in scientific journals that do NOT require pay for publication and do NOT pay the authors to publish. No one pays anyone to publish in scientific journals and those are your primary resources. So... once again knowing what makes something scientific helps you to better understand personalized medicine, medical procedures, treatments, diagnoses and what your doctor is telling you. It is the basis for all of medicine and therefore it is very important.

Conclusion: Putting It All Together

Health is a dynamic, lifelong process shaped by biological, psychological, social, and environmental factors. As I have tried to show in this book, effective healthcare is not limited to the treatment of disease, but involves prevention, informed decision-making, patient engagement, and continuous evaluation of outcomes. True health autonomy can only be achieved through having the right information and being able to ask the right questions. The modern healthcare system is complex and navigating it successfully requires both knowledge and active participation. Patients who understand their conditions, treatment options, and the structure of care delivery are better equipped to engage in shared decision-making, adhere to treatment plans, and recognize when further evaluation or advocacy is necessary. Health literacy is therefore not optional—it is a critical component of safe and effective care.

Health is a complicated issue and involves more than just medicine. Lifestyle factors, access to care, psychosocial stressors, and support systems play a substantial role in both short-term and long-term outcomes. In order to have control over your health, you have to be aware of the things that are included when we say the term "healthcare". Throughout life, health priorities will change. Preventive care, early detection, risk reduction, and chronic disease management each require different approaches and varying levels of medical engagement. Periodic reassessment of health goals and care plans is essential to ensure that interventions remain appropriate, evidence-based, and aligned with your needs and circumstances.

Ultimately, high-quality healthcare is a collaborative process. Clinicians provide expertise and guidance, but patients remain the central decision-makers in their own care. When clinical knowledge, patient values, and systematic follow-up are combined, outcomes improve and care becomes both more effective and more sustainable. The goal is not the unrealistic pursuit of perfect health, but the consistent application of informed, rational, and proactive health decisions over time. This approach supports not only longevity, but also function, quality of life, and overall well-being.

Here's to Love, Life, and the Pursuit of Health!

Everyday Medical Terms Everyone Should Know A pla

A plain-language guide to help patients and families understand common healthcare words.

GENERAL MEDICAL TERMS

Acute: A condition that starts suddenly and usually lasts a short time.

Chronic: A long-term condition that may last months or years.

Benign: Not cancerous

Malignant: Cancerous

Diagnosis: The medical name given to a disease.

Prognosis: The expected outcome or course of a disease. How you will heal, how long it will take etc.

Symptom: Something the patient feels or reports, a subjective feeling, pain is a good example.

Sign: Something a healthcare provider can measure like blood pressure, temperature or pulse rate.

MEDICATIONS & TREATMENT

Prescription (Rx): Medication ordered by a healthcare provider, these have to come from a doctor and you will get them at a pharmacy.

Over-the-Counter (OTC): Medication available without a prescription, like Tylenol or Ibprofen.

Dosage: How much medication to take and how often.

Side Effect: An unintended but common reaction. Something that may happen when you take the medicaion, like being drowsy when you take a   allergy medications.

Adverse Reaction: A harmful or dangerous response. Like being allergice to penicillin or having life threaning reactions to other medications.

Antibiotic: Treats bacterial infections, not viruses.

TESTS & RESULTS

Lab Work : Blood, urine, or other tests that involve bodily fluids.

Imaging: X-ray, CT, MRI, anything that physically takes a "picture" or image of a body part.

Biopsy: Taking a piece of tissue to look at under the microscope, specifically to see if something is cancer or not.

Negative Result: No abnormal findings, normal findings.

Positive Result: Something detected, abnormal result.

VITAL SIGNS

Blood Pressure: Force of blood against artery walls.

Heart Rate: Beats per minute.

Temperature: Body heat; fever $\geq 100.4°F$.

BMI: Body Mass Index, the percentage of fat you have compared to your total body weight.

COMMON CONDITIONS

Inflammation: Redness, swelling, irritation, it is a common body reaction that is supposed to go away but doesn't always.

Infection: Caused by bacteria, viruses, fungi, or parasites.

Autoimmune Disease: Immune system attacks the body.

Allergy: Immune response to a substance that it normally would not respond to, your body overacts to the presence of normal things.

Dehydration: Not enough water.

HEALTHCARE & INSURANCE

Primary Care Provider: Main provider, can be a doctor, nurse practitioner or physcian's assistant.

Specialist: Advanced training in one area, like a cardiologist or psychiatrist.

Referral: Something that your PCP will give a specialist that says you should see them. This should not be confused with prior authorization.

Copay: Fixed visit cost.

Deductible: Paid before insurance coverage.

EMERGENCY TERMS

Emergency: Life-threatening condition.

Stroke: Sudden brain function loss.

Sepsis : An infection that has spread to your whole body usually through your blood.

Shortness of Breath: Difficulty breathing.

GENETIC TERMS

DNA (Deoxyribonucleic Acid): The instruction manual inside your cells. DNA tells your body how to grow, develop, and function.

Chromosome: Packages of DNA found in each cell. Humans usually have 23 pairs (46 total), one from each parent.

Genetic Mutation (Variant, polymorphism): A change in a gene. Some mutations are harmless, some cause disease, and some increase disease risk.

Inherited: A trait or condition passed from parents to children through genes.

Genetic Disorder: A disease caused by changes in genes or chromosomes, not the same thing as hereditary.

Carrier: Someone who has one copy of a gene change but usually does not have symptoms. They can pass it to their children.

Dominant: A genetic trait that only requires one changed gene from one parent to show up.

Recessive: A genetic trait that requires two changed genes (one from each parent) to show up.

Autosomal: A gene located on one of the numbered (non-sex) chromosomes.

X-Linked: A gene located on the X chromosome. These conditions often affect males more severely.

Genetic Testing: A medical test that looks at your DNA to find gene changes.

Family History: Information about diseases that run in your family.

Hereditary Cancer: Cancer caused by inherited gene changes (for example, certain breast or colon cancers).

BRCA Gene: Genes linked to higher risk for breast and ovarian cancer when mutated.

Prenatal Testing: Testing done during pregnancy to check for certain genetic conditions in a baby.

Newborn Screening: Routine testing done shortly after birth to check for treatable genetic conditions.

Genetic Counseling: Meeting with a trained healthcare professional who explains genetic risks and testing options.

Genome: All of a person's DNA combined.

Personalized Medicine (Precision Medicine): Medical care tailored to your genetic makeup.

Trait: A characteristic, like height or hair color, influenced by genes.

Risk Factor: Something that increases the chance of developing a disease (may include genetics).

Epigenetics: Changes in how genes work without changing the DNA itself (can be influenced by environment and lifestyle).

Somatic Mutation: A gene change that happens during a person's lifetime (not inherited).

Chromosomal Abnormality: A change in the number or structure of chromosomes.

Genes: Code that provides instructions for building proteins and determine traits. It is the basic blueprint for your cells.

Genotype: The set of instructions or combination of instructions that make up the blueprint.

Phenotype: The expression of the code (genotype), observable traits and characteristics as defined by that code.

Genome: All of the genes in an organism, all the genes in your body

Genome-Wide Association Study (GWAS): looking at the all the genes (code) and all the phenotypes (expression) of those genes

About the Author

Melissa Paquin, PhD, is a healthcare genetics researcher, educator, and founder of The Progenext Group. Her journey into medicine began in childhood, watching her mother study for nursing school exams—an experience that sparked a lifelong passion for both healthcare and science.

Dr. Paquin earned her Bachelor of Science in Biology from Eastern Connecticut State University, followed by a Master of Science in Biology from the University of Nebraska Kearney. She completed her PhD in Healthcare Genetics at Clemson University's School of Nursing, where her doctoral research focused on the genetic pathways and demographic differences in papillary renal cell carcinoma subtypes, work that directly impacts personalized cancer treatment options.

With over a decade of experience in higher education, Dr. Paquin has taught courses ranging from introductory biology to advanced genetics and healthcare genetics at various academic institutions. Her teaching philosophy centers on making complex scientific concepts accessible and relevant to students' lives; a mission she extends beyond the classroom through *Love, Life, and The Pursuit of Health.*

As a self-described "giant nerd" who took extra science classes in high school simply to learn more, Dr. Paquin has witnessed firsthand the dangerous gap between cutting-edge scientific research, clinical practice, and patient understanding. This gap, which she has seen hurt too many people, inspired her to write this book. Her unique perspective as both a researcher and educator allows her to translate the complex world of genetics, personalized medicine, and evidence-based practice into language that empowers everyday people to take control of their healthcare decisions.

Dr. Paquin lives in Hampton, Georgia, where she continues her work bridging the worlds of science, medicine, and patient advocacy.

She believes that health autonomy is not a luxury but a right—and that it begins with knowledge.

Here's to Love, Life, and The Pursuit of Health!